Princess Fitness

Earn Your Fitness Crown

By: Stephanie Vargas

Princess Fitness

ISBN:0692605584
ISBN-13:9780692605585

ACKNOWLEDGMENTS

To my family, friends, coaches, and mentors that have come into my life and supported, motivated, and pushed me to believe in myself and follow my dreams. Thank you. Being able to share my passion of health, happiness, and loving yourself with not just my community but the world is the best feeling. I hope this book inspires, and builds confidence in women of all ages. Find that Fitness Crown!. Be happy, and love yourself.

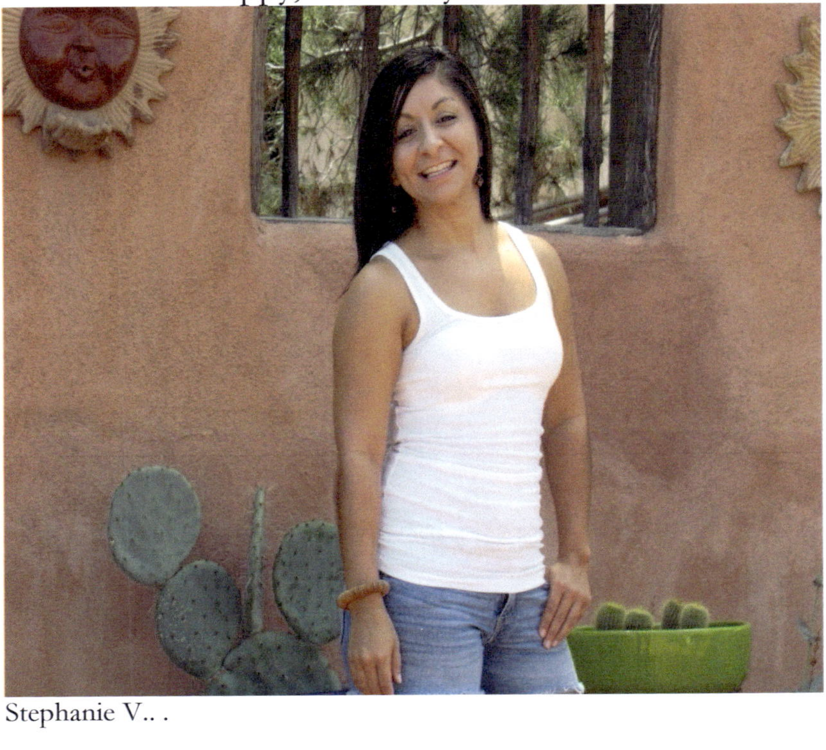

Stephanie V.. .

CONTENTS

1. ***GET FIT LIKE A PRINCESS SHOULD***

Out of all the books on healthy living in all the world you opened mine… Thank you! I know the title "Princess Fitness" can lead to certain mental images that really are not what I am talking about. I would like to share with you what "Princess Fitness" actually means to me. Everyone has their circumstances and situations that can be used as a barrier or a wall to climb. No matter what kind of woman you are or the issues you may face, all women want to be seen and treated like a Princess. Women are now more empowered than ever in history and yet we are still programmed to put everything and everyone before ourselves. Princess Fitness is about giving women the tools to take back your power and make yourself a priority, starting with our bodies and health. We all love to get a compliment; but deep inside we all know there is not a compliment out there that will make you feel as good as when you can fit into those jeans that have been sitting in the back of your closet, or looking at yourself in the mirror and seeing your body with loving eyes rather than critical skepticism. This feeling is not something that can be given, it has to be worked for and earned. What will it take for you to earn your Fitness Crown and feel success and joy?

My name is Stephanie and I am 36 years old, but my motto is “25 for life.” “25 for life,” that’s what I tell people when they ask my age. I have been working with adult and youth fitness for 12 years. I started as a gymnastics coach for girls and I loved it! Being able to see what dedication, hard individual work, and team work can really do is amazing beyond words. I was in the gym one day and I was asked to fill in for an instructor. I side yes without hesitation, not knowing that it was a group of 3 and 4 year olds. From that moment I found my passion, teaching is fun! As I matured and started working more in the fitness world, exercise became a new way of life for me. I wasn't practicing for the big game, but I was learning about my body. What could I do to motivate myself now that I was out of school and no one was telling me to exercise? Running was what I fell into.

I added running to my fitness classes, that I continue to teach, and the lifestyle that emerged has taken me to new heights. I registered for my first half Marathon, 13.1 miles, on an impulse, just because I wanted the challenge. What was I thinking?! This decision turned out to be the beginning of a new life for me. To date I have successfully completed 8 half marathons, 1 full marathon, and I continue to teach fitness classes. I understand my body better, I love teaching fitness classes to adults and kids. My goal in life is to help people live happier and healthier lives. Even with various competitions and classes, running 8 half marathons, and completing my first 26 mile Bataan Death March in Las Cruces, NM, I still had not reached my peak level, what I call the "Fitness Crown."

Earning that Fitness Crown is different for each of us. Just like our bodies are different and we have different goals or aspirations, we will all have different moments that give us that feeling of success and joy … or as I think of it the "Fitness Crown." The day I got my Crown was a random, average day at the gym. I had stared lifting weights, something new for me, and was about four weeks into my program when I was doing my routine and I looked in the mirror…I could see my biceps... I even flexed in the mirror! That was MY First Fitness Crown moment.

"It is NOT my goal to train you until you look like a supermodel or a bodybuilder, but rather to be a healthy, beautiful, woman in your own eyes."

I tell everyone who asks me about my style of training the

above quote. I tell them that their goals are my goals for them, to be healthy. With so many different workout trends there is literally something for everyone. Just as each of us has a different body, you cannot expect the program that your best friend is doing to provide you with the exact same results. Understanding the differences in yourself and accepting them is key to your individual success. Ask yourself; do you do better in a group or one on one? Are you wanting to lose weight or to tone your body? Are you staring a workout for personal reason or did your doctor suggest it? How much time can you make for your body and health?

No one is asking you to compete in the next bikini competition or telling you to give up **all** your favorite foods. My goal is to help you put the wheels in motion and make it your lifestyle. I want to help women be happy and healthy with who they are and help them look in the mirror with pride, loving what they see; Healthy foods give energy, strength, and keep you young at heart and in the mind. A strong mind, body, and soul is essential to any woman who wants to rule their world. We need to put ourselves first in our health and fitness so we can be the leaders in our homes, jobs, and the world around us.

It takes 4 weeks for you to see a change in your body 8

weeks for your friends to notice 12 weeks for the rest of the world to notice: don't quit, give it time.

Changing and breaking habits that we have grown up with take time; but if it does not challenge you, it won't change you. You have to want to make the change. We are only given one body. Take care of it! You can't get a new one. Medical bills and prescriptions are a high price to pay compared to some slight changes in your daily lifestyle now. Believe that you can do it one meal at a time, one workout at a time and each day will add up until one day you don't realize that it's your lifestyle. Remember you are what you eat… DON'T BE FAST, CHEAP, OR FAKE. Remember if it comes out of a drive through window, it's probably not the healthiest meal you could be eating.

80% Nutrition + 20% Exercise = A HEALTHY LIFESTYLE

We live in a fast world and we need to slow down and eat better with fresher, cleaner foods. Learn new ways to make your favorite foods. Portion size is crucial. It's okay to love cake, just remember, you don't have to eat the whole cake when a slice will cure the craving. Add any kind of vegetable to your meals (work your way up to the ones you consider scary), switch ground meat for turkey, AND STOP frying your food. Save the restaurants for special occasions. If you have a crazy busy work schedule, prepare as much of your food on your time off. Prepping your meals will allow you to make “quick meals” healthier than say, having Mac and Cheese.

2. DETOX/CLEANSE

Completing a Detox or Cleanse is a great way to kick off any fitness program or health plan. I always complete a detox or cleanse before starting any training/workout program. If you know you do not make the best food choices (fast food, soda, breads) and you have a goal of weight loss, complete a cleanse/detox so that you can start with a clean slate. These are my top 4 favorite cleanses. I will always encourage you to do your research and do what works for you. Always check with a medical professional before beginning any new health programs, especially if you have pre-existing medical issues.

**Ask your doctor before beginning any new health program, make sure to inform your doctor about any preexisting conditions. **

1) The Cayenne Pepper Cleanse

1 gallon spring water

2 cups fresh squeezed lemon juice

2 cups natural maple syrup

1 1/3 cayenne pepper Tsp

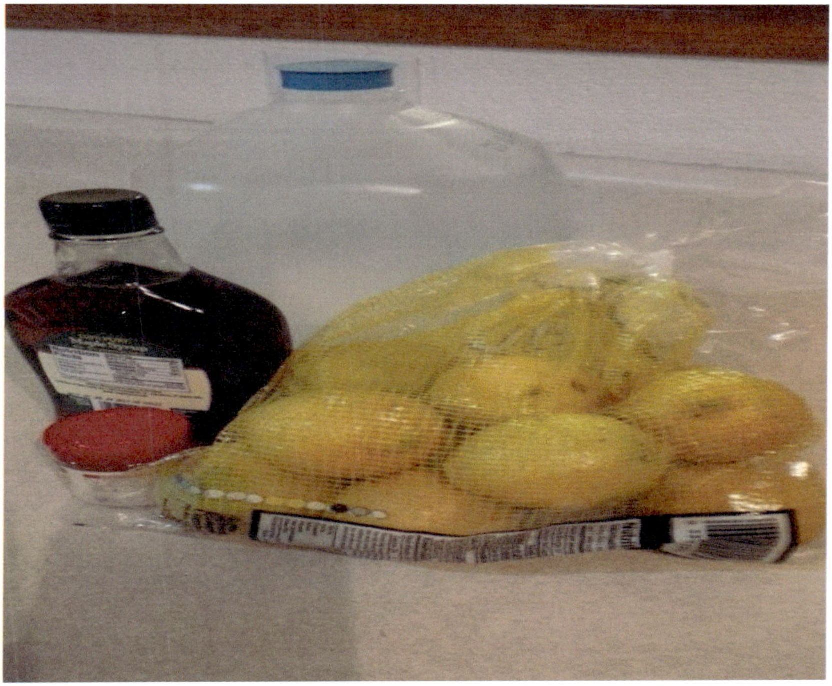

*Lemon juice helps break up fat

*Maple syrup provides the energy

*Cayenne pepper breaks up the dairy

Keep it chilled! This is one drink that is better cold! The real challenge is NOT to eat **AT ALL.** Only drink this mix and water for the first 5 days. Do not workout, just walk if anything. After you finish the first 5 days, keep drinking the mix but introduce ONLY vegetables, fruit, and small amounts of protein back into your diet. After 5 days of this you will add healthy dairy: Low fat milk, yogurt, small amounts of chesses NO bread or Pasta. You should only be drinking the mix before lunch and dinner. Bread and pasta are the last things to put back in. NO white flour of any form, and your water intake should be at least 8 glasses a day by this time. Water and more_Water - not ice tea or lemonade, not juice, not soda, WATER.

2) Apple Cider Vinegar Cleanse

3 cups water

2 tbsp. Apple cider vinegar

1 lemon juiced

1/2 tsp. cinnamon

1/2 tsp. honey

This is best COLD, so I make it the night before and put it in to chill. Drink it first thing, before eating breakfast.

3) Water Detox

1 Jar or Picher

58 ounces spring water

1 grapefruit slice

1 tangerine slice

1 cucumber slice

20 mint leaves

Drink 1 glass of this water mix before each meal. You can continue to add water for up to 5 days, then start a new batch.

4) Warm Coconut Cleanse

1 coffee cup of water

1 spoon full coconut oil

2tbsp lemon juice

2 tbsp. apple cider vinegar

Microwave for about 1minute or use hot water initially. Drink this each morning before eating breakfast.

*With any detox or cleanse your body will flush out the unneeded and sometimes harmful byproducts of the foods we eat. Water is very important when doing these, or any detox/cleanse. It is imperative that you hydrate as this will help your body flush out what your body doesn't need. This is the clean slate and the first step to making a healthier you! Food is fuel for your body, it gives you energy and nutrients. Remember, you are what you eat, so don't be fast, cheap, or fake.

3. ***WATER… WATER… AND MORRE WATER***

We need about 10 glasses of water a day; feeling thirsty doesn't just mean that you need water, it means you've needed it for a while. Thirst is your body's way of saying that it's been too long and you are now dehydrated. One of the early signs of dehydration is a heavy, foggy headache, the kind that makes it hard to think straight. Instead of taking ibuprofen try drinking a glass of water. Hydration is essential to every part of your body. If food is the fuel then water is the lubricant, water keeps everything flowing smoothly. It is easier to keep track of your water intake if you have a water bottle. I'm not suggesting that you go out and buy a specific water bottle but anything that has the amount on it. Get creative!

4. FINDING YOUR PRINCESS WAY

As I have said several times, "We are all different!" What works for one may not work for another. Do what works for you, make your own path and plans to fit your lifestyle. Life is hectic and chaotic and if you have children forget about having any brain juice at the end of the day! If you have children and they are in sports or activities use their practice times to do your workout. Get a group of friends and moms together and while your kids are being healthy you can too! Set an example for your friends and family. Be the trend setter and build that confidence and take control of your body! A key to any workout plan is food. Food is our fuel, without it we are not able to do as much. Slowly incorporate more healthy foods and make better choices in meal times. This takes a little planning, but in the end makes meal time less stressful. Meal planning saves you time and money. If you have kids get them involved in what is being planned.

Sit down with everyone in the household and plan the meals that everyone will eat and enjoy. There will be some moans and groans, but there are a lot of great ideas for healthier versions of the foods you have been eating. Before heading out to the grocery store plan out your week, for example: Monday - grilled chicken, white rice and mixed veggies; do you have all the items or what do you need to purchase? Planning your meals ahead of time allows you to prep and make sure that everything is on hand before it is time to cook and eat. Most of the time you can prepare the majority of the food ahead of time and keep it in the freezer or refrigerator, then it is just preparing the fresh veggies and dinner is served.

We all have our comfort foods. It is no secret that many people are emotional eaters and when the emotions are high, it is never the "healthy" food that gets eaten. Taking a little time to see if there is a healthy alternative to the way you are cooking can make a huge difference in your health. If you are still using Crisco to cook anything, please consider switching to vegetable oil or olive oil to cook with instead. If you are a soda drinker rather than having that second soda have a glass of water.

Jumping from diet to diet isn't healthy for your body; creating healthy eating habits and finding balance is your key. Why be healthy? The answer is simple really, to get the most from your body. You want to live and be happy, it's a basic human desire, do something to help yourself get to that goal. If you are healthy and get hurt, a healthy body will recover faster. A healthy body will also recovery from illness faster and is less likely to get sick when illnesses are cycling; such as the flu or stomach bugs. Being overweight has a lot of risks; diabetes, high blood pressure, heart disease and stroke to name the more severe. Fatigue, low self-esteem, anxiety, depression, sleep apnea, sleep disturbances and irritability are some of the more common effects of living overweight. If you have children, it is important that you know they see you and you are passing these habits on to your kids. New Mexico has a huge number of youth with diabetes and obesity. It takes the whole family to make a change.

As a Hispanic woman, I was taught to show love with food and to eat everything on my plate, otherwise I was being disrespectful and wasteful. If you love someone you want them to be healthy and happy, right? Serve the right portion sizes and more natural foods. I'm not suggesting that you can't eat what you love, but find your balance, find what works for you. I am fortunate enough to live in the Southwest and there is very easy access to various CHILI! I love chili, it is one of the richest sources of vitamins A and

C, capsaicin- the substance that causes your mouth to burn when you eat chili. Capsaicin jump-starts the digestive process, increasing metabolism, and can help keep weight off.

Sometimes we get so busy in our daily lives that we don't eat. Skipping meals is the worst thing you could do to your body. When you skip meals your body goes into a starvation mode where it thinks that it has to store everything. So by not eating, you are telling your body that it cannot depend on a regular fuel supply it starts storing as much as it can to make sure that it keeps running. The kicker of this is that the body is going to store the unhealthy stuff because it can run longer on less which means that your metabolism will slow down and this is the tired that you might be feeling. So, anything that has any fat in it will be stored in your body, usually in the gut area. If you eat consistently throughout the day your body will not need to store up and your metabolism will speed up and the stored fat will gradually dissipate.

5. FOOD AND LIFE

Being from Las Cruces, NM. Spanish rice is one of my favorite dishes to make. Normally you would put oil in the pan and cook the rice. I changed it up a little, I don't add any oil, but I let the rice get nice and brown with the heat and I add a small can of V8 juice instead of tomato sauce. I still season it the same salt, garlic, onion powder, and you would never know the difference. V8 juice is a great alternative to your tomato ingredient.

Calabacitas another of my favorite foods to make and it is super easy and fast. In a pan place squash, green zucchini, corn, tomatoes, and green chile, I add V8 to dish for additional seasoning and sauce, (if wanted to add chicken).

Here is an example of healthy eating for one day:
Remember this is a small book to get the wheels in motion to build a healthier you.

Breakfast-diary, fruit, protein, granola

Snack-dairy and fruit

Lunch- fruit, protein, grain, veggies

Snack- diary and veggies

Dinner- veggies, protein, grain

Breakfast ideas:

Coffee only 2 cups nothing fancy

Hot water, lemon and honey

Green tea, mint and honey

Protein shakes are good and fast

oatmeal hot or cold add fruit, flaxseed, honey

apples, peanut butter and flaxseed

Wheat toast, peanut butter, bananas, honey and flaxseed

yogurt, fruit

protein pancakes with honey and peanut butter

egg whites, asparagus, spinach, cheery tomato's, hot sauce, chili

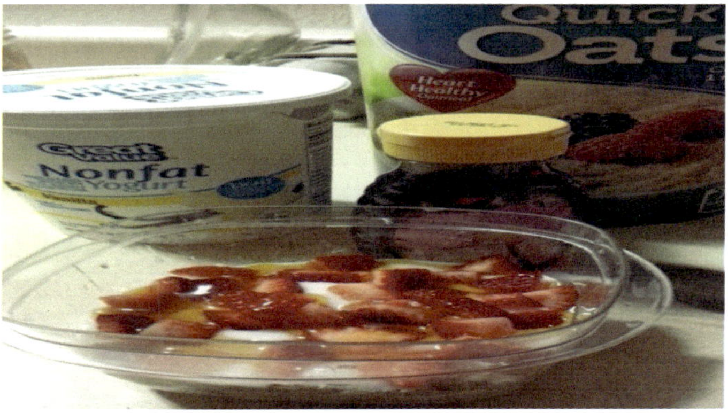

Lunch ideas:

salad with chicken, tuna, fish

tuna, avocado, tomatoes

egg salad eat with celery sticks

half sandwich with soap

turkey slices with cheese 2, cucumbers, carets, avocado and tomato's NO bead

2 boiled eggs with a hand full of asparagus

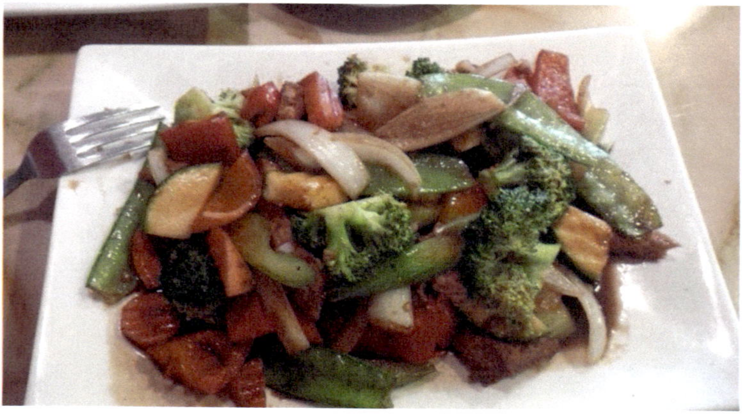

Dinner ideas:

Calabacitas

chicken with rice and veggies

Fish with rice and veggies

veggies soup

ground turkey with beans and green chili

sushi

chicken, red potatoes, carrots, asparagus, broccoli, really any and all the veggies you want

*turkey, chicken and fish

Water - Water and more Water

Snacks are super important for energy throughout the day. Just like everything else in life it is making the decision

that works best for you, not just the fastest or closest option.
Prepare and Plan!

PRINCNESS Workouts

Before starting your workout have a plan. Know what you are doing, what you will need, and have it ready. Get your mind right and focus on what you are about to do. I work on my mind set during my warm up. Remember this is your time, your body, and your workout, NO matter what! If you're with a group, personal trainer, or by yourself you will get what you put into your workout. No matter what your fitness goals are you can always change it up and push yourself.
Some people are old at 18 and some people are young at 90… time is a concept that humans created. Don't be defined by your age! No matter what your mobility level is, there is a program that will help you reach your goal. A little bit goes a long way! Strengthen the muscles and bones to reduce the effects of arthritis and some chronic pain issues. Enable better balance, improved cardiovascular functioning, feel younger every workout, and improve respiratory activity. There are a variety of exercises designed to increase muscular strength, range of motion,

and improved mobility so don't be afraid to try different exercise or class and find what works for you.

**Ask your doctor before beginning any new health program, make sure to inform your doctor about any preexisting conditions. **

6 A SAMPLE WORKOUT PLAN

Warm up - Pick your favorite upbeat, fast paced song and **MOVE** from beginning to end, **DONT STOP**

Pick 4 moves – Do each move 10 times, 10-15 second break, repeat this 3 more times.

Get your Yoga Mat or towel, here come the abs - there are so many choices but pick your favorites and move quickly. Do sets of 10 to 20 of each exercise, using at least 8 different exercise's

Cool down - stretch, breath, and focus on what you just accomplished.

You can utilize all the home equipment that you have purchased over the years. If you have a closet full of home gym equipment use it. Design a workout utilizing what you already have there is no need to purchase any additional equipment. What do you already have in your home that you can use to make you healthier? You don't always need a gym membership to get healthy. We all have fitness equipment at home we swore we would use eventually. But for most people it becomes the clothes hanger or other use it was not intended for. Well it's time to put that to work. Use what you have. You would be amazed that two cans of beans lifted over your head enough times will work your arms. Using a chair against the wall to do dips or standing push ups against the wall can work on the arms, as well even just a little extra activity can make a world of difference.

Living healthy means a longer life to spend with your children, family and friends; but most of all, YOU will have done something to better yourself and your wellbeing.

Some things to remember on your journey:

- Don't know how to use your gym equipment? Ask for help!
- Seniors and all mobility levels can still be healthy! Age is just a number.
- Keep your mind and body strong and sharp!
- Wear appropriate clothing
- Drink a lot of water
- Eat smart! A Clean and portion controlled diet
    - Get a work out buddy or goal. People who have a workout buddy are more likely to follow through. Be accountable.

If you are sick and tired of being sick and tired… this is the way out! There is NO equipment needed, just a little self-motivation, a little space, and 45minutes. Choose where you want to be; at home or at the park. Understand that home can be distracting and gyms are not for everyone so find a local park or place that you feel comfortable and GO FOR IT! Here are some examples of workouts that can be done at home or in a park:

Working out with reps – Reps, or repetitions, are the number of times one motions is completed. For instance, if your goal is to tone and shape your body use light weights and more reps. Repeat your entire workout 4 times. More is better in this method. When you are done with your sets, put weights down and get in some cardio- Toe Taps 20 seconds as fast as you can. Make sure to get your abdominal workout in at the end! Abs are vital to your progress, your core has to be a priority in every workout. It is important to make sure you cool down and stretch otherwise you could be prone to injury and soreness.
If this is your first time with weights start light; 5lbs for 8 reps. (If you need to go lighter on the weight, use weight you are comfortable with but remember to push yourself and keep your heart rate up)

Optional exercises for Reps

-bicep curl and press up to the sky

-triceps

-hold arms out T (count to 8)

-lunges (8 on each leg)

-squats

Timed workout - test your stamina; do the exercise for time 10-20 seconds as fast as you can, no stopping. Work your way up to 60 seconds gradually. Depending on the number of exercises you choose you should be able to repeat the entire sequence 3 times. Make sure to get your Abs workout in at the end! Abs are vital to your progress, your core has to be priority in every workout. Always, always make sure you cool down and stretch otherwise you could be prone to injury.

Optional exercises for timed:

-jumping jacks

-mount climbers

-high knees

-planks

10 - 8 - 6 - reps building strength, do one exercise, with the same amount of weight for 10, 8, 6 reps before moving on to the next exercise do this 3 times.

Before starting any workout make sure to get your heart going and your blood pumping. A short run, cardio, or aerobic workout to start. End each workout with abs and cool down/stretch. Abs are vital to your progress, your core has to be priority in every workout. Make sure you cool down and stretch otherwise you could be prone to injury.

Optional exercises for 10-8-6:

- chest fly's
- curls and press up
- triceps
- one leg lung (do each leg)
- standing abs work - same elbow to knee and
- opposite elbow to knee do this x 3

7. HOME WORKOUT:

Warm up

- Stretch the neck and back thoroughly to prevent straining or injury
- Jumping Jacks
- High knees
- Squats
- Arm circles forward and back

Get your heart rate up with this warm up. Move quickly while making sure you are doing the exercises correctly. If you are not sure if you are doing something correctly, ask for help… Get a mirror to place in front of you so you can see your posture and breathing. Make sure that you are being safe at all times, remember the key here is to be healthy!

Work out in sets of 10 reps, 4 times all the way through

Make sure to move as quickly as you can to keep your heart rate up but if you need to go a little slower until you feel comfortable doing the exercises then go at your own pace.

The key to success if making sure that you are putting everything you can into your workouts. Safety and doing the exercises correctly is the most important aspect of any workout.

- Push-ups
- Plank possession (hold 5sec) bring knee to elbow (opposite)
- Crunches
- Bicycle crunches
- Squat jump

Stretch and cool down

Working out in the PARK: 10 reps 4 times

- Walk 1 lap, fast Jog 1 lap = 2 laps around the park
- Toe taps (find a bench and tap it out)
- Dips (also on the bench)
- Knees to chest (sit on the bench with your legs extended, them bring them as close to your chest as possible.)
- Squats wide legs (until your bum hits the bench then right back up to the standing position.)
- Push-ups hands on bench (DO NOT KISS THE BENCH! Love your body, including our teeth… Safety!)

Jog 2 laps around the park area. Stretch and head home to your healthy dinner! Get your heart rate up and keep it up for the duration of the workout. Move quickly while making sure you are doing the exercises correctly.

Here is a sample calendar for a moderate work-out:

**Ask your doctor before beginning any new health program, make sure to inform your doctor about any preexisting conditions. **

◄	~ Month 2016 ~					April ►
Sun	**Mon**	**Tue**	**Wed**	**Thu**	**Fri**	**Sat**
1 2 miles Speed 3-4.5 Treadmill	**2** REST DAY	**3** 2 miles Speed 3- 4.5 Treadmill	**4** Walk outside 2 miles	**5** 3 miles Speed 3-4.5 treadmill	**6** REST DAY	**7** Walk outside 2 miles
8 2 miles Speed 3-4.5 Treadmill	**9** REST DAY	**10** 2 miles Speed 3- 4.5 Treadmill	**11** Walk outside 2 miles	**12** 3 miles Speed 3-4.5 Treadmill	**13** REST DAY	**14** Walk outside 2 miles
5 miles peed 3-4.5 readmill	**16** REST DAY	**17** 2 miles Speed 3-4.5 Treadmill	**18** 3 miles Speed 3- 4.5 Treadmill	**19** Walk outside 2 miles	**20** REST DAY	**21** 2 miles Speed 3-4.5 Treadmill
2 miles peed 4.5-5 readmill	**23** REST DAY	**24** 2 miles Speed 4.5-5 Treadmill	**25** 3 miles Speed 4.5-5 Treadmill	**26** 2 miles OUTSIDE	**27** REST DAY	**28** 4 miles OUTSIDE
miles UTSIDE	**30** REST DAY	**31** 3 miles OUTSIDE	**Notes: if you are a first time runner we want to start on the treadmill; find your pace, breathing in through the nose and out thought the mouth.** **Water, healthy eating, and stretching are strongly recommended** **2 rest days only and always walk like you need to get somewhere**			

8 Rest and Sleep

Remember your body needs time to rest and recover. This time will allow your body rebuild itself. When planning a workout, give yourself 3 rest days. 3 days of a hard workouts, pushing yourself. Sweat, Breathe, Clear your mind and smile. Be active, this is great for family time and getting everyone involved. Try running, hiking, swimming, Play with your kids like going outside for walk or going to the park. Keep your body moving and doing different things so you don't get bored and your body keeps changing, getting stronger. The more movement you incorporate into your life the more energy you will produce.

Sleep is an important part that we tend to take for granted. This is when your body can recharge, just like your cell phone, 8 hours of straight sleep. Life circumstances do not always allow for this much consecutive sleep. If you have children or are working multiple jobs you will not get 8 hours of uninterrupted sleep. Do your best! Make a conscious effort to **put down the electronics,** maybe you don't go out with friends tonight after work, remember change will change you and the people closest to you. Try to get as much sleep as you possibly can and work toward a goal of getting 8 hours sleep. If you are working out give yourself two rest days but not in a row, you want to keep the momentum. My days to rest are Monday and Friday because you never know what will happen on those days with my life. Tuesday, Wednesday and Thursday I work hard on myself and make sure that my workouts count. Saturday and Sunday I do something fun; biking, hiking, and swimming, anything that I can do with friends and family. It's also a good time to try a class.

9.*__TIME AND ENERGY__*

When did we stop moving? LIFE! **We have to be just as important to ourselves as others are to us, BE KIND TO YOURSELF**. Children are little balls of energy and sometimes you wonder how they keep going but it boils down to the fact that they are healthy, happy, and active. As adults we have stopped moving, time passed and we became more involved in phones, computers, TV, video games, and work. We have stopped moving, disconnecting from our bodies and our natural way of being. Our body needs to sweat, move, and pump blood to our brain, heart, lungs and muscles. Remember what it feels like to play... kids don't think about how many calories they burn or if they are toning up. No, they just play to play and be happy which keeps them healthy and active. As adults, we need to find what does that for us. Break the routine of life and start doing something active that you find enjoyable. It can be anything from jumping on a trampoline, swimming or hopscotching down the sidewalk. Anything that is out of your normal, is active, and fun- PLAY! PLAYING with kids at a park, don't miss out on the fun by working or being on your phone. The more you move the more energy you will have to do more things and start putting this lifestyle in motion. Remember what it is to smile, be grateful, happy, and look forward to waking up the next day.

10 ***WRAPPING UP***

Motivation is different for each of us. Finding it and using it is the challenge. You can make change on any level and still move forward. When we get stuck in a routine or in a specific way of thinking, it is time for a change. Change in any form is difficult and creates feelings of unease, but any change worth making is worth the anxiety. Do something for yourself. You need to be your own biggest fan and cheerleader. Remember always that you are a strong, independent, beautiful woman and the only person that can take that away, is you. Take your power back and make yourself a priority. You don't have to make huge, sudden changes to be healthier, you just have to believe that you can change. One foot in front of the other and before you know it you are moving forward. Remember, odds are, you have someone looking up to you and you may not even know it. Changing negative habits is not only good for your health, but for the people around you. BREATHE, DRINK WATER, AND STAY IN MOTION!

Remember, every Princess needs a crown! Get started and find your "Fitness Crown!"

Notes:

Workout Journal:

Food Journal:

Made in the USA
Monee, IL
05 November 2026

67378014R00026